W9-BEI-720

THE SEVEN PILLARS *of* HEALTH

50-DAY JOURNAL

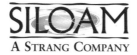

SILOAM

A STRANG COMPANY

Most STRANG COMMUNICATIONS/CHARISMA HOUSE/SILOAM/FRONTLINE/ REALMS products are available at special quantity discounts for bulk purchase for sales promotions, premiums, fund-raising, and educational needs. For details, write Strang Communications/Charisma House/Siloam/ FrontLine/Realms, 600 Rinehart Road, Lake Mary, Florida 32746, or telephone (407) 333-0600.

THE SEVEN PILLARS OF HEALTH 50-DAY JOURNAL by Don Colbert, MD
Published by Siloam
A Strang Company
600 Rinehart Road
Lake Mary, Florida 32746
www.siloam.com

International Standard Book Number: 978-1-59979-203-3

Neither the publisher nor the author is engaged in rendering professional advice or services to the individual reader. The ideas, procedures, and suggestions in this book are not intended as a substitute for consulting with your physician. All matters regarding your health require medical supervision. Neither the author nor the publisher shall be liable or responsible for any loss or damage allegedly arising from any information or suggestion in this book.

While the author has made every effort to provide accurate telephone numbers and Internet addresses at the time of publication, neither the publisher nor the author assumes any responsibility for errors or for changes that occur after publication.

07 08 09 10 11 — 9 8 7 6 5 4 3 2 1
Printed in the United States of America

HOW TO USE THIS BOOK

Welcome to *The Seven Pillars of Health 50-Day Journal*! Just as *The Seven Pillars of Health* main book is broken into fifty days of reading, so is this journal organized for you to complete in fifty straight days with the book. This journal gives the support and accountability you need to make necessary changes in your diet, health, and lifestyle. So, let's get started!

First Step: Assessment and Goals

Before jumping into the daily routine of this journal, it's important to assess your current health status and establish personal goals. What concerns do you carry about your health right now? What results do you hope to see after fifty days of learning and applying these important pillars of health to your life? A place to respond to these questions has been provided on pages 5–7.

Action Steps

After completing each day's reading in the main book, flip to the corresponding day in this journal to find out your action step for the day. These action steps serve as small, daily assignments that integrate the information you've learned with your practical life. A place has been provided on each page to confirm that you've completed the action step for the day.

Make It Personal

This section does what it says: makes the process personal. It offers anywhere from two to four questions each day that make the reading personal *to you*—your own life and habits.

Daily Checkup

The Daily Checkup section helps distill the priorities of the current pillar into a few short questions you'll answer each day of that week. It also provides a daily rating scale to rate your progress each day, plus a space to record additional thoughts as needed.

Weekly Update

Weekly updates afford a chance to check in on your goals, your overall health, and your continuous integration of the previous pillars into your daily life. This is the place to reflect on how you're carrying your new health habits through from week to week.

Final Step: Assessment and Goals

At the end of the fifty-day program, you'll get to evaluate your progress, celebrate the goals you reached, and determine new steps to continue your road toward lifelong health.

FIRST STEP:
ASSESSMENT AND GOALS

Health concerns I have faced in the past five years:

- Cancer
- Diabetes
- Heart disease
- Thyroid disorders
- Asthma
- Irritable bowel syndrome
- High blood pressure
- High cholesterol
- Headaches
- Back pain
- Muscle pain
- Arthritis
- Osteoporosis
- Prostate disorders
- Memory loss
- Insomnia
- Weight gain
- Weight loss
- Eating disorders
- Heartburn and indigestion
- Autoimmune disease
- Chronic fatigue syndrome
- Fibromyalgia

☐ PMS or hormone imbalance

☐ Depression

☐ Other(s): _____

What advice or concerns, if any, has my doctor voiced about my health in the past five years?

_____

_____

_____

_____

What changes in health are most important to me right now?

_____

_____

_____

_____

What factors provide the greatest motivation as I undertake this fifty-day program?

☐ I want to feel better physically.

☐ I want to have more energy.

☐ I want to improve immediate health concerns in my life.

☐ I want to lose weight.

☐ I want to be more active in my lifestyle.

☐ I want to see my kids and grandkids grow up.

☐ I want to break the cycle of my bad habits.

☐ I want to overcome generational health problems in my family.

☐ I want to extend the length and quality of my days.

☐ I want to be a better steward of the body God gave me.

I want to demonstrate better self-control (a fruit of the Spirit) in my life.

I want to spend less money on medical bills.

My current weight: _____
My weight goal: _____

My current blood sugar level: _____
My blood sugar goal: _____

My current blood pressure: _____ / _____
My blood pressure goal: _____ / _____

My current cholesterol level: _____
My cholesterol level goal: _____

In summary, my goals for this fifty-day program are:

_____

_____

_____

_____

_____

_____

_____

_____

_____

DAY 1

Points to Ponder

Water is the single most important nutrient for our bodies and is considered a "miracle cure" for many health conditions. It is involved in every function of our bodies. Your body loses about two quarts of water a day through perspiration, urination, and exhalation. If you wait until you are thirsty to drink water, then you are most likely already dehydrated.

Action Step

Instead of reaching for a soft drink or tea today, drink clean, natural water. Completed?   Yes   No

Make It Personal

How often do I drink water? _____

_____

What other beverages do I usually consume?

_____

_____

_____

What are the reasons I drink water in my daily life?

 Habit
 Thirst
 Exercise
 I like the taste
 I know I'm supposed to
 I don't drink it
 Other: _____

How likely is it that I'm living in a mildly dehydrated state?
 Very likely   It's possible   Doubtful   Definitely not, as I keep myself well hydrated with water every day

Daily Checkup

My daily water intake:

☐ ☐ ☐ ☐ ☐ ☐ ☐ ☐   (one checkbox per 16-ounce bottle)

Other nonwater products I drank today:_____

_____

My Seven Pillars progress today was:
☐ Great   ☐ Good   ☐ Fair   ☐ Poor

My Daily Journal:

_____

_____

_____

_____

_____

_____

_____

_____

_____

_____

_____

_____

_____

_____

Recharge Your Thoughts

Drinking sufficient amounts of the right kinds of water will do more to improve your health than anything else you can do.

DAY 2

Points to Ponder

Dehydration robs from certain areas of the body to keep the brain, heart, lungs, liver, and kidneys well hydrated. Many symptoms of disease are the first sign of the body needing adequate amounts of water. Some of the symptoms of inadequate water intake may include headaches, back pain, joint aches, dry skin, allergies, heartburn, constipation, and memory loss.

Action Step

Stop by the doctor's office or drugstore pharmacy to have your blood pressure taken. Completed? ▢ Yes ▢ No

Today's blood pressure reading: _____ / _____

Make It Personal

Which adverse conditions of dehydration do I already suffer from?

▢ Joint pain and arthritis
▢ High blood pressure
▢ Digestion problems
▢ Asthma

What other physical ailments of mine (headaches, backaches, memory loss, etc.) might be caused by dehydration but relieved with greater water intake? _____

_____

_____

_____

Prior to today's reading, how aware was I of my body's need for water in its daily processes and functions? _____

_____

_____

Daily Checkup

My daily water intake:

☐ ☐ ☐ ☐ ☐ ☐ ☐ ☐   (one checkbox per 16-ounce bottle)

Other nonwater products I drank today: _____

_____

My Seven Pillars progress today was:
☐ Great   ☐ Good   ☐ Fair   ☐ Poor

My Daily Journal

_____

_____

_____

_____

_____

_____

_____

_____

_____

_____

_____

_____

_____

_____

Recharge Your Thoughts

*You are valuable; take care of yourself
and properly hydrate your body.*

DAY 3

Points to Ponder

Water is a powerful nutrient to slow the aging process and to maintain your brain and memory. Your brain cells are mainly water—about 85 percent—and your brain is constantly active, even during sleep. Therefore, your brain needs to be well hydrated.

Action Step

Instead of applying antiaging skin creams or other treatments today, drink extra water. Completed?　☐ Yes　☐ No

Make It Personal

What attempts have I already made (skin creams, pills, spa treatments, etc.) to maintain the youthful look of my skin?

_____

_____

_____

What areas of my body reveal that my skin is likely suffering a lack of hydration? _____

_____

_____

_____

How does my skin look and feel in those areas? _____

_____

_____

_____

In what ways have I noticed my memory slowing? _____

_____

_____

_____

Daily Checkup

My daily water intake:

☐ ☐ ☐ ☐ ☐ ☐ ☐ ☐   (one checkbox per 16-ounce bottle)

Other nonwater products I drank today: _____

_____

My Seven Pillars progress today was:
☐ Great   ☐ Good   ☐ Fair   ☐ Poor

My Daily Journal

_____

_____

_____

_____

_____

_____

_____

_____

_____

_____

_____

_____

_____

_____

Recharge Your Thoughts

Water is the single best beauty treatment on the planet. It keeps your skin supple, your eyes bright, and your body spry.

DAY 4

Points to Ponder

It's best not to drink water straight from the faucet, because tap water may contain toxins, heavy metals, pesticides, residual personal care products, bacteria, and other microbes. One of the chemicals added to our tap water is fluoride. Generally, there are two types of fluoride: the type added to toothpaste (sodium fluoride) and the type added to drinking water (sodium silicofluoride). The latter is the most toxic of the two.

Action Step

Check your city's water supply today. Log on to www.ewg.org/tapwater/findings.php. Click the tab labeled "Local Findings." Select the state and city name to generate a local water system report. Completed? ▢ Yes ▢ No

Make It Personal

When do I usually drink or use tap water? _____

_____

_____

_____

What have I already been doing to avoid contaminants in my water?

_____

_____

_____

_____

How willing am I to purchase a water or shower filter for my home?

_____

_____

_____

Daily Checkup

My daily water intake:

■ ■ ■ ■ ■ ■ ■ ■ (one checkbox per 16-ounce bottle)

Other nonwater products I drank today: _____

_____

My Seven Pillars progress today was:
■ Great ■ Good ■ Fair ■ Poor

My Daily Journal

_____

_____

_____

_____

_____

_____

_____

_____

_____

_____

_____

_____

_____

_____

Recharge Your Thoughts

Water rejuvenates your skin, making you look years younger.

DAY 5

Points to Ponder

Some bottled waters contain more toxins than tap water and are not as closely regulated as tap. If you drink bottled water, check if the manufacturer of the bottled water is a member of the IBWA (International Bottled Water Association). Always properly store your bottled water. Keep it away from chemicals, and store it in a refrigerator if possible. If the container is plastic, check the expiration date or bottling date.

Action Step

Find out if the brands of water you drink belong to the International Bottled Water Association. Log on to www.bottled water.org. Click on "What Is IBWA?" and then "Brand List." Completed?   Yes   No

Make It Personal

What brands of bottled water do I usually drink? _____

_____

_____

Given the list in Appendix C, which bottled water brands available in my area might be wiser choices? _____

_____

_____

How many of these bottled water practices do I already perform?

- Use plastic bottles only once.
- Drink water within a few months of its bottling date.
- Store bottles in the refrigerator.
- Store bottles in dark, cool places.
- Store bottles away from household or industrial chemicals.

Daily Checkup

My daily water intake:

☐ ☐ ☐ ☐ ☐ ☐ ☐ ☐   (one checkbox per 16-ounce bottle)

Other nonwater products I drank today:_____

_____

My Seven Pillars progress today was:

☐ Great   ☐ Good   ☐ Fair   ☐ Poor

My Daily Journal

_____

_____

_____

_____

_____

_____

_____

_____

_____

_____

_____

_____

_____

_____

Recharge Your Thoughts

By giving your body the water it needs, you will maintain your youth and smarts longer.

DAY 6

Points to Ponder

Filtered water is one of the best waters for your body. When choosing a filter, remember that carbon filters are the "entry-level" type of filter and the least expensive. Distilled water and reverse-osmosis water are the purest water. However, they are also the most acidic. In my opinion, alkaline water filters are one of the best types of filters because our bodies thrive best in an alkaline environment, which helps our systems function at an optimum level.

Action Step

Purchase pH strips at the local drugstore to test the pH level of your urine and your bottled water's alkalinity. Completed?   Yes   No

Make It Personal

What type of water filter am I able to purchase right now?

_____

What are the pros and cons of this kind of filter?

Pros: _____

_____

_____

Cons: _____

_____

_____

What can I do to compensate for the cons on this list (take mineral supplements, cut spending in other areas to make up for the expense, etc.)? _____

_____

_____

_____

Daily Checkup

My daily water intake:

☐ ☐ ☐ ☐ ☐ ☐ ☐ ☐   (one checkbox per 16-ounce bottle)

Other nonwater products I drank today: _____

_____

My Seven Pillars progress today was:

☐ Great   ☐ Good   ☐ Fair   ☐ Poor

My Daily Journal

_____

_____

_____

_____

_____

_____

_____

_____

_____

_____

_____

_____

_____

_____

Recharge Your Thoughts

Using a water filter in your home can be a big step toward restoring health to your drinking water.

DAY 7

Points to Ponder

Don't wait until you are thirsty to drink water. If you wait until you're thirsty, you've waited too long. You're probably already dehydrated. Drink at least two quarts of clean water per day. Drink thirty minutes before meals or two hours after meals. Try not to drink excessive amounts of water past 7:00 p.m. Doing so may interfere with your sleep.

Action Step

As a beverage choice at meals, stick to four to eight ounces of room-temperature water. Completed?   Yes   No

Make It Personal

How much water should I drink each day?

_____ ÷ 2 = _____ ounces per day
My weight in pounds

What sources of caffeine do I drink regularly? _____

_____

_____

Do I drink caffeine in moderation?   Yes   No

When do I usually drink beverages, and how much?

_____

_____

How can I adjust my beverage routine to better reflect the guidelines given in today's reading? _____

_____

_____

Daily Checkup

My daily water intake:

▨ ▨ ▨ ▨ ▨ ▨ ▨ ▨   (one checkbox per 16-ounce bottle)

Other nonwater products I drank today: _____

_____

My Seven Pillars progress today was:
▨ Great ▨ Good ▨ Fair ▨ Poor

My Daily Journal

_____

_____

_____

_____

_____

_____

_____

_____

_____

_____

_____

_____

_____

_____

Recharge Your Thoughts

Water is the first and most important pillar upon which to build a healthy life.

WEEKLY UPDATE

General

What positive changes did I notice in my overall health this week?

_____

_____

_____

_____

_____

_____

My weight update: _____

My blood sugar update: _____

My blood pressure update: _____ / _____

My cholesterol level update: _____

Pillar 1: Water

How many ounces of water did I average per day this week?

■ ■ ■ ■ ■ ☐ ☐ (one checkbox per 16-ounce bottle)

What adjustments to my beverage intake do I want to make in the coming week? _____

_____

_____

_____

_____

DAY 8

Points to Ponder

A good night's sleep restores, repairs, and rejuvenates your body. Sleep is important because it is vital for your immune system and your overall health. Sleep also slows down the aging process. Lack of adequate sleep increases your risk of developing type 2 diabetes as well as a host of other diseases.

Action Step

Make sure you get seven to nine hours of sleep tonight.
Completed?   Yes   No

Make It Personal

How many hours of sleep do I currently average each night?

_____

What is my normal bedtime? _____

_____

How important have sleep and rest been in my life?

_____

_____

_____

_____

What effects has a lack of sleep had on my life, either in past experience or presently? _____

_____

_____

_____

_____

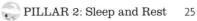

Daily Checkup

Hours I slept last night: _____

My sleep rating: ░ Great ░ Good ░ Fair ░ Poor

Factors that contributed to my good or poor night's sleep:

_____

_____

_____

My Seven Pillars progress today was:
░ Great ░ Good ░ Fair ░ Poor

My Daily Journal

_____

_____

_____

_____

_____

_____

_____

_____

_____

_____

_____

_____

Recharge Your Thoughts

Getting the adequate amount of sleep is beneficial to you, and it benefits those around you.

DAY 9

Points to Ponder

Insomnia affects many people, robbing them of sleep—and, in the long run, good health. Some causes of insomnia are stress, anxiety, depression, chronic pain, caffeine, and medications. Be careful not to eat sugary or high-processed foods before bedtime because they may cause low blood sugar, which makes it difficult for you to sleep.

Action Step

Go for a brisk walk in the afternoon or early evening (at least three hours before bedtime) to prepare your body for more restful sleep tonight. Completed?   Yes   No

Make It Personal

What thoughts usually keep me awake at night? _____

_____

_____

_____

_____

How comfortable are my pillows, mattress, and sheets? _____

_____

_____

_____

What other factors sometimes keep me from a good night's sleep?

_____

_____

_____

_____

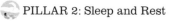

Daily Checkup

Hours I slept last night: _____

My sleep rating: ▢ Great ▢ Good ▢ Fair ▢ Poor

Factors that contributed to my good or poor night's sleep:

_____

_____

_____

My Seven Pillars progress today was:
▢ Great ▢ Good ▢ Fair ▢ Poor

My Daily Journal

_____

_____

_____

_____

_____

_____

_____

_____

_____

_____

_____

_____

Recharge Your Thoughts

When you sleep, your body rejuvenates itself.

DAY 10

Points to Ponder

As a nation we have become too dependent upon energy drinks and medications to keep us awake longer. We need to realize that when we cheat the body from getting the sleep it needs, we may eventually suffer the consequences healthwise. There are stages to our sleep cycle, with stages three and four being the most restful part of sleep. Dreams are important to restore the mind.

Action Step

Sit on a comfortable chair in a darkened room for at least five minutes. If you fall asleep, you may be sleep deprived.

Completed?   Yes   No

Did you fall asleep?   Yes   No

Make It Personal

Do I need an alarm clock to wake up in the morning?
Yes   No

Do I get drowsy while driving short distances or while waiting at traffic lights?   Yes   No

Do I run out of steam in the middle of the day?   Yes   No

Am I irritable and agitated?   Yes   No

Am I a light sleeper who wakes up easily at every noise?
Yes   No

Am I unable to get persistent worries out of my mind?   Yes   No

What are recurring themes or images in my dreams? _____

_____

How do these themes or images reflect my real life, thoughts, and concerns? _____

_____

Daily Checkup

Hours I slept last night: _____

My sleep rating: ▢ Great ▢ Good ▢ Fair ▢ Poor

Factors that contributed to my good or poor night's sleep:

_____

_____

_____

My Seven Pillars progress today was:
▢ Great ▢ Good ▢ Fair ▢ Poor

My Daily Journal

_____

_____

_____

_____

_____

_____

_____

_____

_____

_____

_____

Recharge Your Thoughts

Dreams connect us with our internal intelligence, our true selves, our souls. They are images that have the ability to bring wellness and wholeness.

DAY 11

Points to Ponder

Maintaining a bedtime ritual is essential to a good night's sleep for children *and* adults. Exercise is one way to improve the quality of your sleep. However, exercising within three hours of sleep may interfere with sleep because exercise raises the levels of stress hormones. Eat a light bedtime snack. (See the suggested list on page 50.) Corral your thoughts, and take time to relax.

Action Step

Fill out the appreciation list on page 124.
Completed? ▊ Yes ▊ No

Make It Personal

What activities do I usually engage in from the time I get home from work until the time I go to bed (include times)?

_____

_____

_____

_____

_____

_____

How can I adjust this routine so it better prepares my body and mind for a good night's sleep? _____

_____

_____

_____

_____

_____

Daily Checkup

Hours I slept last night: _____

My sleep rating: ▓ Great ▓ Good ▓ Fair ▓ Poor

Factors that contributed to my good or poor night's sleep:

_____

_____

_____

My Seven Pillars progress today was:
▓ Great ▓ Good ▓ Fair ▓ Poor

My Daily Journal

_____

_____

_____

_____

_____

_____

_____

_____

_____

_____

_____

_____

Recharge Your Thoughts

God designed us to fall asleep when it is dark and to wake up when the sun rises.

DAY 12

Points to Ponder

Your bedroom is a place to retreat, relax, revive, and rejuvenate. For a more sleep-conducive environment, try the following: keep the room dark, filter out noise, get a good mattress and pillow, and make sure the room temperature is comfortable. Pleasure reading or watching TV is acceptable, provided they help you (and your spouse) relax and do not add stress.

Action Step

Eliminate light from shining through your bedroom window at night, and keep the room dark. Completed?   Yes   No

Make It Personal

Which of the following items do I currently keep in my bedroom?
- Night-light
- Computer
- Television
- Work-related paperwork
- Piles of books
- Other hobbies and/or projects

What can I do to make my bedroom feel more like a sleep haven?

_____

_____

_____

_____

Which of these things will I commit to doing this week?

_____

_____

_____

_____

Daily Checkup

Hours I slept last night: _____

My sleep rating: ▢ Great ▢ Good ▢ Fair ▢ Poor

Factors that contributed to my good or poor night's sleep:

_____

_____

_____

My Seven Pillars progress today was:
▢ Great ▢ Good ▢ Fair ▢ Poor

My Daily Journal

_____

_____

_____

_____

_____

_____

_____

_____

_____

_____

_____

_____

Recharge Your Thoughts

Your bedroom should look like an inviting place of rest.

DAY 13

Points to Ponder

Some people rely on sleep medications, whether over the counter or prescribed, which may become addictive and disrupt their natural sleep cycle. Yet nature has provided sleep aids without adding the side effects of prescription medications. Although these sleep aids, such as valerian, 5-HTP, calcium, melatonin, magnesium, L-theanine, and bedtime teas, are natural products, always consult with your health care provider before taking them, especially if you are pregnant, nursing, or taking prescription medications. Some supplements may interfere with certain medications.

Action Step

Drink a cup of bedtime herbal tea before bed tonight.
Completed?　　Yes　　No

Make It Personal

What sleep aids (if any) have I used in the past?_____

_____

_____

What factors kept me from sleeping well at that time? _____

_____

_____

_____

_____

What methods have I found most effective for helping me sleep well in the night? _____

_____

_____

_____

Daily Checkup

Hours I slept last night: _____

My sleep rating: ▢ Great ▢ Good ▢ Fair ▢ Poor

Factors that contributed to my good or poor night's sleep:

_____

_____

_____

My Seven Pillars progress today was:
▢ Great ▢ Good ▢ Fair ▢ Poor

My Daily Journal

_____

_____

_____

_____

_____

_____

_____

_____

_____

_____

_____

_____

Recharge Your Thoughts

The very best sleep aid is the Word of God. It puts all things in perspective and offers perfect peace.

DAY 14

Points to Ponder

One of the most basic principles is a day of rest. Take time to rest. For many, rest may mean going out for lunch or dinner, watching a good movie, or spending time with family and friends. Rest, however, does not mean cooking, cleaning house, or working in the yard.

Action Step

Take a break this afternoon for a ten- to thirty-minute power nap. Completed?　Yes　No

Make It Personal

What activities promote a sense of well-being and rest in my body, mind, and spirit? _____

_____

_____

_____

_____

If I had one day of rest each week, what would I choose to do on that day? _____

_____

_____

_____

_____

What would it take to incorporate this day of rest into my schedule?

_____

_____

_____

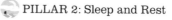

Daily Checkup

Hours I slept last night: _____

My sleep rating: ▓ Great ▓ Good ▓ Fair ▓ Poor

Factors that contributed to my good or poor night's sleep:

_____

_____

_____

My Seven Pillars progress today was:
▓ Great ▓ Good ▓ Fair ▓ Poor

My Daily Journal

_____

_____

_____

_____

_____

_____

_____

_____

_____

_____

_____

_____

Recharge Your Thoughts

A Sabbath rest humbles us by reminding us that, after all is said and done, God is the source of our strength.

WEEKLY UPDATE

General

What positive changes did I notice in my overall health this week?

_____

_____

_____

_____

My weight update: _____

My blood sugar update: _____

My blood pressure update: _____ / _____

My cholesterol level update: _____

Pillar 1: Water

How many ounces of water did I average per day this week?

◼ ◼ ◼ ◻ ◻ ◻ ◻   (one checkbox per 16-ounce bottle)

What adjustments to my beverage intake do I want to make in the coming week? _____

_____

_____

_____

Pillar 2: Sleep and Rest

How many hours of sleep did I average per night this week? _____

What adjustments to my sleep routine do I want to make in the coming week? _____

_____

_____

_____

DAY 15

Points to Ponder

No more living on the "SAD" diet. It's time to start choosing living foods over dead foods. Remember that from the time we start eating until the time the food reaches our small intestines, it takes twenty minutes for leptin to signal the brain to stop eating.

Action Step

Eat a salad with lots of greens and vegetables in it today.
Completed?   Yes   No

Make It Personal

What living foods are already a regular part of my diet?

_____

_____

_____

_____

What dead foods do I eat on a regular basis? _____

_____

_____

_____

_____

What will be the greatest challenge for me in choosing living foods over dead foods this week? _____

_____

_____

_____

_____

Daily Checkup

Living foods I ate today: _____

_____

_____

_____

Dead foods I ate today: _____

_____

_____

_____

My Seven Pillars progress today was:
 Great Good Fair Poor

My Daily Journal

_____

_____

_____

_____

_____

_____

_____

_____

_____

_____

Recharge Your Thoughts

Living foods (such as fruits, veggies, and whole grains) will always be healthier for you than processed foods.

DAY 16

Points to Ponder

There are many reasons why Americans can't lose weight and keep it off; however, the main reason is that dead foods give comfort. Emotions are usually at the root of an obesity problem. However, you can exercise self-control and retrain yourself not to turn to food for comfort. You need to learn how to forgive yourself and not burden your mind with guilt and shame.

Action Step

Read and sign the Agreement to Lose Weight on page 125. Completed? ■ Yes ■ No

Make It Personal

Which of the "bad food" cycles do I commonly fall into?

_____

_____

_____

In what specific ways has my body seen the effects of poor food choices? _____

_____

_____

_____

What spiritual and emotional triggers are likely at the root of my poor food choices? _____

_____

_____

_____

_____

Daily Checkup

Living foods I ate today: _____

_____

_____

_____

Dead foods I ate today: _____

_____

_____

_____

My Seven Pillars progress today was:
■ Great   ■ Good   ■ Fair   ■ Poor

My Daily Journal

_____

_____

_____

_____

_____

_____

_____

_____

_____

_____

Recharge Your Thoughts

You have been given the power to restrain yourself by having the ability to control your cravings. You make the choice.

DAY 17

Points to Ponder

Ask yourself this question: *What would Jesus eat?* God's initial design was for man to be a vegetarian. However, we are no longer under the law but under grace. Every creature of God is good as long as it is received with thanksgiving.

Action Step

Use the chart on page 126 to calculate your body mass index (BMI). Completed?　Yes　No

Which category do you fall into right now?
　Underweight　Normal　Overweight　Obese

Make It Personal

How important a part has meat played in the diet I've been maintaining? _____

_____

_____

_____

In what ways, if any, does this need to change? _____

_____

_____

_____

How does Paul's exhortation that "all things are permissible but not all things are beneficial" apply to my life? _____

_____

_____

_____

_____

Daily Checkup

Living foods I ate today: _____

_____

_____

_____

Dead foods I ate today: _____

_____

_____

_____

My Seven Pillars progress today was:
　Great　　Good　　Fair　　Poor

My Daily Journal

_____

_____

_____

_____

_____

_____

_____

_____

_____

_____

Recharge Your Thoughts

We are supposed to be "living epistles." Others should look at us and visibly see a difference, not only in our attitude but also in our very appearance, which begins with what we eat.

DAY 18

Points to Ponder

Stay on the lighter side of life by enjoying living foods. The more processed a food is and the more sugar and toxic fats a food contains, the more harm it will do to your body. Limit your intake of fatty meats such as bacon, hot dogs, sausage, and cold cuts.

Action Step

Purchase a box of stevia to replace aspartame and Splenda as a sweetener in your diet. Completed? ▓ Yes ▓ No

Make It Personal

What "Franken-foods" have got me addicted? _____

_____

_____

_____

_____

In what ways does refined sugar reign in my diet? _____

_____

_____

_____

_____

What can I do to reduce the amount of fast food I consume?

_____

_____

_____

_____

_____

Daily Checkup

Living foods I ate today: _____

_____

_____

_____

Dead foods I ate today: _____

_____

_____

_____

My Seven Pillars progress today was:
  Great   Good   Fair   Poor

My Daily Journal

_____

_____

_____

_____

_____

_____

_____

_____

_____

_____

Recharge Your Thoughts

Those who choose "life-giving" foods go on to live long and healthy lives.

DAY 19

Points to Ponder

Fruits, vegetables, whole grains, and healthy oils are all "living food." Not all fats are bad. In fact, your body needs good fat. Good alternatives are extra-virgin olive oil, almonds, macadamia nuts, and flaxseeds. Depending on the oil, you can lightly stir-fry your food. Never deep-fry.

Action Step

Check the glycemic index of a variety of foods you normally eat. Log on to www.glycemicindex.com and click on "GI Database." Completed? Yes No

Make It Personal

Approximately how many servings of fruits and vegetables am I eating each day? _____

_____

_____

Which fruits, vegetables, and other living food recommendations in this chapter would I like to increase in my diet? _____

_____

_____

_____

How will I go about making organic, whole grain, and nonpreservative foods a more substantial part of my diet? _____

_____

_____

_____

_____

Daily Checkup

Living foods I ate today: _____

_____

_____

_____

Dead foods I ate today: _____

_____

_____

_____

My Seven Pillars progress today was:
▢ Great ▢ Good ▢ Fair ▢ Poor

My Daily Journal

_____

_____

_____

_____

_____

_____

_____

_____

_____

_____

Recharge Your Thoughts

*It's time to make over your pantry and fridge with living foods
so you can look and feel your best!*

DAY 20

Points to Ponder

Foods that we used to think were good for us, in reality may be making us toxic and causing diseases, such as many of our fish and charred hamburgers and steaks. When choosing meats, choose the leanest cuts of free-range or grass-fed meats. Avoid irradiated meats; know the symbol for irradiated meats. Dark chocolate is very high in antioxidants; however, make sure it has low sugar and no vegetable oils. Avoid milk chocolate.

Action Step

Purchase a half gallon of organic skim milk to replace your usual milk this week. Completed?　　Yes　　No

Make It Personal

What kind of meat do I normally eat, and in what contexts (broiled, grilled, fast food, deep-fried, etc.)? _____

_____

_____

_____

What are the sources of dairy in my diet? _____

_____

_____

_____

How do I need to change my eating habits with meat and dairy?

_____

_____

_____

_____

Daily Checkup

Living foods I ate today: _____

_____

_____

_____

Dead foods I ate today: _____

_____

_____

_____

My Seven Pillars progress today was:
　Great 　Good 　Fair 　Poor

My Daily Journal

_____

_____

_____

_____

_____

_____

_____

_____

_____

_____

Recharge Your Thoughts

Once you start buying the right kinds of meats and preparing them in a healthy way, you can fully enjoy them as part of your regular diet.

DAY 21

Points to Ponder

What cookware you use to cook your food is just as important as how you cook it. Use CorningWare, glass, or stainless-steel cookware when cooking. When eating, take time to chew your food instead of eating quickly. Eating too quickly sends the wrong signals to your body. Chew each bite twenty to thirty times, and set your fork down between bites. Plan your meals, cook healthy, and most of all, enjoy the company of your family or friends.

Action Step

Pay attention today to how many chews you normally take before swallowing food. Work up to chewing each bite at least twenty to thirty times by the end of the day. Completed?   ▉ Yes   ▉ No

How many chews did you average at first? _____

Make It Personal

What fresh foods do I often buy and store for long periods of time—past their actual point of freshness? _____

_____

_____

How do I normally prepare my vegetables (boiling, microwaving, grilling, steaming, deep-frying, etc.)? _____

_____

_____

How can I do this more healthfully? _____

_____

How do I need to adjust the cookware I use for preparing food?

_____

_____

Daily Checkup

Living foods I ate today: _____

_____

_____

_____

Dead foods I ate today: _____

_____

_____

_____

My Seven Pillars progress today was:
☐ Great ☐ Good ☐ Fair ☐ Poor

My Daily Journal

_____

_____

_____

_____

_____

_____

_____

_____

_____

_____

Recharge Your Thoughts

A fresh-made dish is more nutritious than one you cook and refrigerate.

WEEKLY UPDATE

General

What positive changes did I notice in my overall health this week?

_____

_____

_____

_____

My weight update: _____

My blood sugar update: _____

My blood pressure update: _____ / _____

My cholesterol level update: _____

Pillar 1: Water

How many ounces of water did I average per day this week?

☐ ☐ ☐ ☐ ☐ ☐ ☐ (one checkbox per 16-ounce bottle)

What adjustments to my beverage intake do I want to make in the coming week? _____

_____

_____

_____

Pillar 2: Sleep and Rest

How many hours of sleep did I average per night this week? _____

What adjustments to my sleep routine do I want to make in the coming week? _____

_____

_____

_____

Pillar 3: Living Foods

How did I excel in choosing living foods this week? _____

_____

_____

_____

How did I depend upon dead foods? _____

_____

_____

What adjustments to my eating habits will I make in the coming week? _____

_____

_____

DAY 22

Points to Ponder

Like water, when our bodies are stagnant, they become a breeding ground for disease. It's time to stir the waters of your life again and begin exercising. Exercise refreshes your body, renews your energy, and gives you strength.

Action Step

Take a 10–15 minute walk today. Completed?   Yes   No

Make It Personal

How am I stirring the waters right now in my life? _____

_____

_____

_____

_____

_____

Which of my usual activities promote stagnation? _____

_____

_____

_____

_____

_____

What keeps me from exercising? _____

_____

_____

_____

_____

_____

Daily Checkup

Today I stirred the waters by: _____
_____
_____
_____
_____

My Seven Pillars progress today was:
☐ Great   ☐ Good   ☐ Fair   ☐ Poor

My Daily Journal

_____
_____
_____
_____
_____
_____
_____
_____
_____
_____
_____
_____
_____

Recharge Your Thoughts

Exercise refreshes your body and clears it of toxins and cellular garbage, sharpening your mind and giving you strength and energy.

DAY 23

Points to Ponder

Exercise helps to prevent many diseases and keep excess weight off. It improves the immune system, helps to maintain normal blood pressure, conditions the heart, and prevents heart disease. Exercise also helps control blood sugar in diabetics and improves lymphatic flow, which helps remove cellular waste.

Action Step

Purchase a pedometer. Wear it each day to monitor your usual activity level and to work toward increasing your average daily step count. Completed?   Yes   No

Make It Personal

What health problems do I fear may become a reality for me in the future? _____

_____

_____

_____

_____

_____

Why are these health problems potential realities for me (current activity level, family history, etc.)? _____

_____

_____

_____

_____

_____

_____

Daily Checkup

Today I stirred the waters by: _____

_____

_____

_____

_____

My Seven Pillars progress today was:
Great   Good   Fair   Poor

My Daily Journal

_____

_____

_____

_____

_____

_____

_____

_____

_____

_____

_____

_____

_____

Recharge Your Thoughts

Your body was designed to move.

DAY 24

Points to Ponder

Exercise tones the muscles, improves digestion, promotes frequent bowel movements, slows down the aging process, promotes mental health, and even improves the memory. Done correctly, exercise will help you sleep better.

Action Step

Stop by a sporting goods store to find a good pair of walking shoes. Completed?　■ Yes　■ No

Make It Personal

What forms of exercise have I enjoyed in the past? _____

_____

_____

_____

_____

What did I enjoy about those exercise routines? _____

_____

_____

_____

_____

How can I incorporate a similar enjoyment of exercise now?

_____

_____

_____

_____

_____

Daily Checkup

Today I stirred the waters by: _____

_____

_____

_____

_____

My Seven Pillars progress today was:
 Great Good Fair Poor

My Daily Journal

_____

_____

_____

_____

_____

_____

_____

_____

_____

_____

_____

_____

_____

Recharge Your Thoughts

*A walking routine is a good foundation for a
lifetime of exercise.*

DAY 25

Points to Ponder

Walking is one of the safest and easiest forms of aerobic exercise. Walk slow enough so that you can talk, but fast enough so that you can't sing. Never exercise along a busy highway where toxic fumes and automobile exhaust can put your health at risk. When beginning an exercise program, begin with a low-intensity activity and gradually increase your level. Warm up five minutes before exercising by walking slowly, and take five minutes after exercising to cool down.

Action Step

Get in touch with a friend who can be your exercise partner or provide accountability. Completed? ▓ Yes ▓ No

Who will be your partner? _____

Make It Personal

What is my target heart rate?

$$220 - \underline{\qquad} = \underline{\qquad}$$
My age   Gauge number

$$\underline{\qquad} \times .6 = \underline{\qquad}$$
Gauge number   Low target

$$\underline{\qquad} \times .9 = \underline{\qquad}$$
Gauge number   High target

What aerobic exercise routine will I commit to? _____

_____

_____

What exercise locations are best for me? _____

_____

_____

Daily Checkup

Today I stirred the waters by: _____

_____

_____

_____

_____

My Seven Pillars progress today was:
▨ Great ▨ Good ▨ Fair ▨ Poor

My Daily Journal

_____

_____

_____

_____

_____

_____

_____

_____

_____

_____

_____

_____

_____

Recharge Your Thoughts

Simply moving more during the day will enable you to reap the tremendous benefits of exercise.

DAY 26

Points to Ponder

Weight training and calisthenics are part of a holistic approach to exercise, plus they help to build strong bones and muscles. Stretching promotes flexibility and can also serve as a good warm-up prior to exercise. Perform repetitions slowly using good technique.

Action Step

Practice the postural and flexibility stretch at least three times today. (See pages 134–135 of the main book.) Completed?　　Yes　　No

Make It Personal

What weight-training or calisthenic exercises can I begin to do to strengthen my bones and muscles? _____

_____

_____

_____

Which of the weightlifting benefits do I most desire to experience? (See page 133 of the main book.) _____

_____

_____

In what areas of my body do I want to build muscular strength using heavier weights with low repetitions? _____

_____

_____

In what areas of my body do I want to simply tone my muscles using lighter weights with high repetitions? _____

_____

_____

Daily Checkup

Today I stirred the waters by: _____

_____

_____

_____

_____

My Seven Pillars progress today was:
■ Great   ■ Good   ■ Fair   ■ Poor

My Daily Journal

_____

_____

_____

_____

_____

_____

_____

_____

_____

_____

_____

_____

_____

_____

Recharge Your Thoughts

From age thirty on, everyone needs to exercise either with weights or calisthenics to keep their muscles and bones strong.

DAY 27

Points to Ponder

There are many alternatives to traditional exercises. Yoga is a healthy alternative to more traditional means of exercise. It combines low-impact exercise with stretching and breathing. Tai Chi involves slow, smooth movements. It's great for older people, especially those who suffer from arthritis. Tai Chi movements help improve muscle mass, strength, and flexibility, among its other many health benefits. Pilates also involves low-intensity exercise with stretching. It helps reduce stress, increase flexibility, and tone muscles. Ballroom dancing is a fun way to exercise without feeling as if you are exercising. It's a great way for couples to reconnect and spend time together.

Action Step

Contact your local community college, vocational school, or community activity center to find out when their next dance or alternative exercise class begins. Completed?　Yes　No

Make It Personal

What alternative forms of exercise have I enjoyed in the past?

_____

_____

_____

What did I enjoy about them? _____

_____

_____

What appeals to me about the alternative forms of exercise listed here? _____

_____

_____

_____

Daily Checkup

Today I stirred the waters by: _____

_____

_____

_____

_____

My Seven Pillars progress today was:
☐ Great   ☐ Good   ☐ Fair   ☐ Poor

My Daily Journal

_____

_____

_____

_____

_____

_____

_____

_____

_____

_____

_____

_____

_____

Recharge Your Thoughts

*Though the body doesn't like being exercised at first,
after about three weeks it will change its mind:
it will desire and expect to exercise.*

DAY 28

Points to Ponder

Building an exercise program into your schedule doesn't have to be boring; it can be as fun as you make it. Find exercises that you enjoy doing—such as swimming or dancing. Look for opportunities throughout the day to fit in occupational/transportation or "leisure-time" activities such as gardening, walking the dog, parking your car in the space furthest away from the door to the store, taking the stairs instead of the elevator, and so on. Be creative and innovative with your exercise routine, and make it an exercise program for life!

Action Step

Park your car at the far end of the parking lot today, and take the stairs whenever possible. Completed?   Yes   No

Make It Personal

How can I best build exercise into my schedule? _____

_____

_____

_____

Which routine activities are part of my daily life? (See pages 142–143 in the main book.)

Activity: _____   Calories burned per hour:_____

Activity: _____   Calories burned per hour:_____

Activity: _____   Calories burned per hour:_____

Activity: _____   Calories burned per hour:_____

Given my usual participation in these routine activities, how many calories do I likely burn on a daily basis? _____

_____

_____

Daily Checkup

Today I stirred the waters by: _____
_____
_____
_____
_____

My Seven Pillars progress today was:
■ Great ■ Good ■ Fair ■ Poor

My Daily Journal

_____
_____
_____
_____
_____
_____
_____
_____
_____
_____
_____
_____
_____
_____

Recharge Your Thoughts

Seize every opportunity to increase your activity level.

WEEKLY UPDATE

General

What positive changes did I notice in my overall health this week?

_____

_____

_____

_____

My weight update: _____

My blood sugar update: _____

My blood pressure update: _____ / _____

My cholesterol level update: _____

Pillar 1: Water

How many ounces of water did I average per day this week?

☐ ☐ ☐ ☐ ☐ ☐ ☐ (one checkbox per 16-ounce bottle)

What adjustments to my beverage intake do I want to make in the coming week? _____

_____

_____

_____

Pillar 2: Sleep and Rest

How many hours of sleep did I average per night this week? _____

What adjustments to my sleep routine do I want to make in the coming week? _____

_____

_____

_____

Pillar 3: Living Foods

How did I excel in choosing living foods this week? _____

_____

_____

_____

How did I depend upon dead foods? _____

_____

_____

_____

What adjustments to my eating habits will I make in the coming week? _____

_____

_____

_____

Pillar 4: Exercise

What victories did I have in stirring the waters this week?

_____

_____

_____

How will I continue to build up my regular exercise schedule in the coming week? _____

_____

_____

_____

DAY 29

Points to Ponder

Toxicity permeates our environment, which is affecting our health, but there are some things we can change. The toxic levels in our air, water, and food supply are increasing annually. There is hope through detoxifying our waste management system.

Action Step

Use pH strips to check your pH level at the start of each day this week. Completed?   Yes   No

Make It Personal

What have I previously learned about toxins in the environment?

_____

_____

_____

_____

_____

What methods of detoxification have I heard about before?

_____

_____

_____

_____

What products in my home likely have chemicals and toxic fillers in them? _____

_____

_____

_____

_____

Daily Checkup

My pH level today was: _____

I avoided exhaust and secondhand smoke today: Yes   No

I perspired today: Yes   No

My Seven Pillars progress today was:
    Great   Good   Fair   Poor

My Daily Journal

_____

_____

_____

_____

_____

_____

_____

_____

_____

_____

_____

_____

_____

_____

_____

_____

Recharge Your Thoughts

There are simple things you can start doing today to rid your body of toxins and to help your waste management systems keep them out.

DAY 30

Points to Ponder

Breathing in secondhand smoke for an hour is worse than actually smoking four cigarettes yourself. Practically all nonorganically grown produce is tainted with pesticides and herbicides. Our food supply may contain parasites from workers not washing their hands.

Action Step

Wash your bed sheets in hot water to eliminate dust mites. Completed? ▪ Yes ▪ No

Make It Personal

Which air hazards like smog, exhaust, cigarette smoke, forest fires, and others make an impact on my daily life? _____

_____

_____

_____

_____

What food products are regular sources of toxins for me? (See pages 152–155 in the main book.) _____

_____

_____

_____

_____

How can I go about reducing my toxic intake from food?

_____

_____

_____

Daily Checkup

My pH level today was: _____

I avoided exhaust and secondhand smoke today: ▢ Yes ▢ No

I perspired today: ▢ Yes ▢ No

My Seven Pillars progress today was:
▢ Great ▢ Good ▢ Fair ▢ Poor

My Daily Journal

_____

_____

_____

_____

_____

_____

_____

_____

_____

_____

_____

_____

_____

_____

_____

Recharge Your Thoughts

Doing something as simple as taking a few slow, deep breaths will enable you to unwind and secrete adequate amounts of digestive enzymes and hydrochloric acid.

DAY 31

Points to Ponder

Mercury, found in most dental fillings, is one of the most toxic elements on the planet. Some vaccinations, such as the DT booster and flu vaccine, still contain mercury. Silver fillings are composed of about 50 percent mercury. A common ingredient used in perfumes and colognes is toluene, which may cause heart arrhythmias and nerve damage. Armed with the correct knowledge, you can begin to reclaim your health from unexpected sources of toxins.

Action Step

Make an appointment with your doctor to have a heavy metal screen completed. Completed?　Yes　No

Make It Personal

How many silver amalgam fillings are in my mouth? _____

Which household cleaners do I use on a regular basis?

_____

_____

_____

What personal care products do I use on my body each day?

_____

_____

_____

How can I reduce the use of chemicals in my home and on my body? _____

_____

_____

_____

Daily Checkup

My pH level today was: _____

I avoided exhaust and secondhand smoke today: ☐ Yes ☐ No

I perspired today: ☐ Yes ☐ No

My Seven Pillars progress today was:
☐ Great ☐ Good ☐ Fair ☐ Poor

My Daily Journal

_____

_____

_____

_____

_____

_____

_____

_____

_____

_____

_____

_____

_____

_____

_____

_____

Recharge Your Thoughts

Aerobic exercise can increase lymphatic flow threefold, which means that the body can release three times the amount of toxins with regular aerobic exercise.

DAY 32

Points to Ponder

Toxins may trigger most degenerative diseases, including cancer and heart disease. Body odor is sometimes a sign of a toxic body. Pesticides and solvents, such as cleansers, are fat soluble and are stored in fatty tissues, including tissues in the brain, breasts, and prostate gland.

Action Step

Purchase a pair of rubber gloves to use when cleaning the house with chemical solvents. Completed?   Yes   No

Make It Personal

What symptoms of toxic overload do I already experience? (See page 164 in the main book.) _____

_____

_____

_____

Which toxic triggers in my life are likely the primary causes of these symptoms? _____

_____

_____

_____

What alternative choices can I make to avoid these toxins?

_____

_____

_____

_____

_____

Daily Checkup

My pH level today was: _____

I avoided exhaust and secondhand smoke today:　Yes　No

I perspired today:　Yes　No

My Seven Pillars progress today was:
　Great　Good　Fair　Poor

My Daily Journal

_____

_____

_____

_____

_____

_____

_____

_____

_____

_____

_____

_____

_____

_____

_____

_____

Recharge Your Thoughts

As you help your body take out the trash, your body will begin to heal itself.

DAY 33

Points to Ponder

Your body's waste management system was designed to take out the toxic trash on a daily basis, not once a week. Get adequate amounts of fiber on a daily basis (about twenty-five to thirty grams a day). Limit your intake of meat and dairy; always choose the leanest cuts of meat and fat-free or low-fat organic dairy products. Eat organic foods as often as possible, and remember, the thicker the peel in nonorganic produce, the safer it is, generally speaking.

Action Step

Circle all the alkaline foods on pages 170–171 of the main book that you are likely to eat. Add a handful of these foods to this week's shopping list. Completed? ■ Yes ■ No

Make It Personal

How often do I expel food from my system? _____

_____

_____

What sources of fiber are already in my diet? _____

_____

_____

How can I include more fiber, if necessary? _____

_____

_____

What foods on the acidifying food list do I need to reduce in my diet? (See page 171.) _____

_____

_____

_____

Daily Checkup

My pH level today was: _____

I avoided exhaust and secondhand smoke today: ▢ Yes ▢ No

I perspired today: ▢ Yes ▢ No

My Seven Pillars progress today was:
▢ Great ▢ Good ▢ Fair ▢ Poor

My Daily Journal

_____

_____

_____

_____

_____

_____

_____

_____

_____

_____

_____

_____

_____

_____

_____

_____

_____

Recharge Your Thoughts

Your body is designed with an incredible defense system that keeps you healthy even under extreme circumstances.

DAY 34

Points to Ponder

Perspiration is another way to rid the body of toxins. Sweating is actually a sign of being healthy. Don't be afraid to perspire when you exercise; it generally means you are healthy!

Action Step

Buy a loofah sponge or natural soft-bristle brush to start a regular dry-skin brushing routine. Completed? ☐ Yes ☐ No

Make It Personal

How often do I perspire? ☐ Often ☐ Sometimes ☐ Never

What activities make me sweat? _____

_____

_____

_____

_____

_____

What can I do to increase my perspiration level to better detoxify through my skin? _____

_____

_____

_____

_____

How can I take better care of my "third kidney," the skin?

_____

_____

_____

Daily Checkup

My pH level today was: _____

I avoided exhaust and secondhand smoke today: ☐ Yes ☐ No

I perspired today: ☐ Yes ☐ No

My Seven Pillars progress today was:
☐ Great ☐ Good ☐ Fair ☐ Poor

My Daily Journal

_____

_____

_____

_____

_____

_____

_____

_____

_____

_____

_____

_____

_____

_____

_____

Recharge Your Thoughts

By sweating and taking care of your skin you help your body get rid of toxins.

DAY 35

Points to Ponder

Periodic fasting is one of the most powerful ways to detoxify the body. Consider having indoor plants or an air purifier for your home. Choose natural cleansers instead of chemical boxed cleansers.

Action Step

Purchase an inexpensive air purifier for your bedroom.
Completed?   Yes   No

Make It Personal

What air hazards do I need to guard against or investigate in my home? _____

_____

_____

_____

Which organic cleansers would be useful alternatives for my lifestyle? _____

_____

_____

_____

What steps can I take to incorporate one day of fasting into my life each month? _____

_____

_____

_____

_____

Daily Checkup

My pH level today was: _____

I avoided exhaust and secondhand smoke today: ▢ Yes ▢ No

I perspired today: ▢ Yes ▢ No

My Seven Pillars progress today was:
▢ Great ▢ Good ▢ Fair ▢ Poor

My Daily Journal

_____

_____

_____

_____

_____

_____

_____

_____

_____

_____

_____

_____

_____

_____

_____

_____

Recharge Your Thoughts

Our world is toxic, but you don't have to be. You can decrease your exposure and risk by making choices that help your body's elimination systems take out the toxic trash.

WEEKLY UPDATE

General

What positive changes did I notice in my overall health this week?

_____

_____

_____

_____

My weight update: _____

My blood sugar update: _____

My blood pressure update: _____ / _____

My cholesterol level update: _____

Pillar 1: Water

How many ounces of water did I average per day this week?

☐ ☐ ☐ ☐ ☐ ☐ ☐ (one checkbox per 16-ounce bottle)

What adjustments to my beverage intake do I want to make in the coming week? _____

_____

Pillar 2: Sleep and Rest

How many hours of sleep did I average per night this week? _____

What adjustments to my sleep routine do I want to make in the coming week? _____

_____

Pillar 3: Living Foods

How did I excel in choosing living foods this week? _____

_____

_____

How did I depend upon dead foods? _____

_____

_____

What adjustments to my eating habits will I make in the coming
week? _____

_____

_____

Pillar 4: Exercise

What victories did I have in stirring the waters this week?

_____

_____

How will I continue to build up my regular exercise schedule in
the coming week? _____

_____

_____

Pillar 5: Detoxification

How did I help my body detoxify this week? _____

_____

_____

How can I continue to detoxify and reduce toxic exposure in the
coming week? _____

_____

_____

DAY 36

Points to Ponder

Whole grains such as barley, millet, oats, and brown rice contain more of the nutrients we need than their refined counterparts, such as white rice or white bread. Proper digestion is essential to helping the body absorb the nutrients our bodies need. However, even the healthiest diet needs to be supplemented with nutrients.

Action Step

Help digestive enzymes break down your food by drinking minimal fluids with meals and chewing your food thoroughly today. Completed?　Yes　No

Make It Personal

What vitamins or other nutritional supplements have I taken in the past? _____

_____

_____

_____

How frequently did I take them? _____

_____

_____

What was my motivation for taking them? _____

_____

_____

_____

What effects did they have on my body and sense of well-being?

_____

_____

_____

Daily Checkup

Supplements I took today:

- Whole-food multivitamin
- Phytonutrient powder
- Omega-3 supplement
- Sublingual B_{12}
- Digestive enzyme
- Other:_____

Foods on the phytonutrient rainbow I ate today (see pages 206–211 in the main book):

- Red: _____
- Red/purple: _____
- Orange: _____
- Orange/yellow: _____
- Yellow/green: _____
- Green: _____
- White/green: _____

My Seven Pillars progress today was:
- Great   Good   Fair   Poor

My Daily Journal

_____

_____

_____

Recharge Your Thoughts

As we come under God's grace, He has blessed us with the tools and the knowledge that will make our land—and our food— rich in nutrients again.

DAY 37

Points to Ponder

A healthy diet will rarely supply all the nutrients you need. In fact, most Americans don't get even basic amounts of recommended vitamins and minerals. Nutrients that are commonly lacking in the American diet include vitamins A, B_6, C, D, E, and K, magnesium, calcium, fiber, and potassium.

Action Step

Add two foods from each food chart to your grocery list this week. Completed?   Yes   No

Make It Personal

Based on the food charts in this chapter, which vitamins and minerals are abundantly present in my diet already? _____

_____

_____

_____

_____

Which ones do I need to receive more often? _____

_____

_____

_____

What foods will I eat to increase the presence of these vitamins and minerals in my body? _____

_____

_____

_____

_____

Daily Checkup

Supplements I took today:

- Whole-food multivitamin
- Phytonutrient powder
- Omega-3 supplement
- Sublingual B$_{12}$
- Digestive enzyme
- Other:_____

Foods on the phytonutrient rainbow I ate today (see pages 206–211 in the main book):

- Red: _____
- Red/purple: _____
- Orange: _____
- Orange/yellow: _____
- Yellow/green: _____
- Green: _____
- White/green: _____

My Seven Pillars progress today was:
- Great - Good - Fair - Poor

My Daily Journal

_____

_____

_____

Recharge Your Thoughts

Vitamins and minerals are at the very foundation of your health.

DAY 38

Points to Ponder

Antioxidants are to free radicals what water is to a raging forest fire burning out of control. The key antioxidants that our bodies produce include glutathione, superoxide dismutase, and catalase. Five antioxidants that work as a team include vitamin C, vitamin E (all eight forms), coenzyme Q_{10}, lipoic acid, and glutathione. Carnosine is a nutrient that can also act as a powerful antioxidant.

Action Step

Spend 5–10 minutes in the sun without sunblock today to increase your vitamin D intake. (Don't forget to wear sunglasses.) Completed?　Yes　No

Make It Personal

What types of food, diseases, injuries, and/or toxic exposures are likely sources of free radicals in my life? (See page 199 in main book.) _____

_____

_____

_____

Which living food antioxidants do I consume on a regular basis to fight my free-radical exposure? (See list on page 204 in main book.) _____

_____

_____

_____

_____

Daily Checkup

Supplements I took today:

- Whole-food multivitamin
- Phytonutrient powder
- Omega-3 supplement
- Sublingual B_{12}
- Digestive enzyme
- Other:_____

Foods on the phytonutrient rainbow (pages 206–211 in the main book) I ate today:

- Red: _____
- Red/purple: _____
- Orange: _____
- Orange/yellow: _____
- Yellow/green: _____
- Green: _____
- White/green: _____

My Seven Pillars progress today was:

Great   Good   Fair   Poor

My Daily Journal

_____
_____
_____

Recharge Your Thoughts

Antioxidants are the most important key to the free radical riddle.

DAY 39

Points to Ponder

Phytonutrients give fruits and vegetables their color. Fruits and vegetables can be grouped according to color and provide a rainbow of health, protecting us from cancer and heart disease. Red—tomatoes, watermelon—contain lycopene. Red/purple—blueberries, grapes—contain a powerful flavonoid called anthocyanidin. Orange—carrots, cantaloupes, sweet potatoes—contain carotenoids. Orange/yellow—oranges, tangerines—contain bioflavonoids. Yellow/green—spinach, mustard greens—contain lutein. Green—broccoli, cabbage—are cruciferous vegetables containing multiple powerful phytonutrients, especially DIM and indole-3-carbinole. White/green—onions, garlic—contain quercetin.

Action Step

Pick up a week's supply of organic blueberries—a powerful berry high in ORAC units. Completed?　▢ Yes　▢ No

Make It Personal

Why phytonutrient benefits are important to me? _____

_____

_____

What colors of the phytonutrient rainbow do I consume most regularly? _____

_____

_____

How can I increase my intake of the other colors of the rainbow?

_____

_____

_____

Daily Checkup

Supplements I took today:

- Whole-food multivitamin
- Phytonutrient powder
- Omega-3 supplement
- Sublingual B_{12}
- Digestive enzyme
- Other:_____

Foods on the phytonutrient rainbow I ate today (see pages 206–211 in the main book):

- Red: _____
- Red/purple: _____
- Orange: _____
- Orange/yellow: _____
- Yellow/green: _____
- Green: _____
- White/green: _____

My Seven Pillars progress today was:

Great   Good   Fair   Poor

My Daily Journal

_____

_____

_____

Recharge Your Thoughts

Phytonutrients are hard at work in your body, saving you from various threats you probably were never even aware of.

DAY 40

Points to Ponder

Do any of the supplements you are currently taking contain the toxic fillers or agents mentioned in today's entry? Supplements, like prescription medications, have become a multibillion-dollar business. Recommended amounts of nutrients don't tell you how much you need to be healthy, but how much you need to prevent disease. *Caveat emptor*—let the buyer beware: there are supplements that may be harming you, such as rancid fish oils.

Action Step

Stop by your local smoothie or health food shop today for a shot of wheatgrass juice—an excellent source of amino acids, vitamins, minerals, and essential fatty acids. Completed?   Yes   No

Make It Personal

What has hindered me from taking supplements on a regular basis?

_____

_____

_____

_____

How have I used nutrition labels to help me select food products?

_____

_____

_____

What caution do I need to take in reading labels now?

_____

_____

_____

Daily Checkup

Supplements I took today:

- Whole-food multivitamin
- Phytonutrient powder
- Omega-3 supplement
- Sublingual B_{12}
- Digestive enzyme
- Other: _____

Foods on the phytonutrient rainbow I ate today (see pages 206–211 in the main book):

- Red: _____
- Red/purple: _____
- Orange: _____
- Orange/yellow: _____
- Yellow/green: _____
- Green: _____
- White/green: _____

My Seven Pillars progress today was:

- Great   Good   Fair   Poor

My Daily Journal

_____

_____

_____

Recharge Your Thoughts

Supplementation should never be random, but well researched, thought out, and tailored to your specific condition and needs.

DAY 41

Points to Ponder

Supplements do not exist to replace a healthy diet; they exist to complement it. Taking supplements in high doses or taking an excessive amount of supplements can actually harm you. Generally, the unhealthiest patients that I see are the ones who are mega-dosing.

Action Step

Pick something on which you have a tendency to "mega-dose" and take a breather from it this week. Completed?   Yes   No

What did you choose? _____

Make It Personal

In what ways can I relate to the man in the story at the beginning of the chapter? _____

_____

_____

_____

What has motivated my engagement in harmful mega-dosing behavior before? _____

_____

_____

How can I ensure that I keep a proper balance between supplementation and healthy lifestyle and dietary choices?

_____

_____

_____

Daily Checkup

Supplements I took today:

- Whole-food multivitamin
- Phytonutrient powder
- Omega-3 supplement
- Sublingual B$_{12}$
- Digestive enzyme
- Other: _____

Foods on the phytonutrient rainbow I ate today (see pages 206–211 in the main book):

- Red: _____
- Red/purple: _____
- Orange: _____
- Orange/yellow: _____
- Yellow/green: _____
- Green: _____
- White/green: _____

My Seven Pillars progress today was:

Great   Good   Fair   Poor

My Daily Journal

_____

_____

_____

Recharge Your Thoughts

As long as you eat a healthy diet, you don't have to meet all your nutritional needs with supplements.

DAY 42

Points to Ponder

Everyone needs a good multivitamin and a phytonutrient supplement. Most everyone needs essential fats in the form of high-grade fish oil. If you are over fifty years of age, you will also need extra antioxidants, extra calcium and vitamin D, a sublingual B_{12}, and maybe a digestive enzyme and/or HCL.

Action Step

Pick up a supply of whole-food multivitamins, high quality omega-3 supplements, and phytonutrient powder at the health store today to begin proper supplementation. Completed?   Yes   No

Make It Personal

Why does Dr. Colbert recommend a whole-food multivitamin, an omega-3 supplement, and a phytonutrient powder as the foundation for supplementation? _____

_____

_____

_____

_____

_____

How has my perspective on nutritional supplements changed or broadened over the course of this week's pillar? _____

_____

_____

_____

_____

_____

Daily Checkup

Supplements I took today:

- Whole-food multivitamin
- Phytonutrient powder
- Omega-3 supplement
- Sublingual B$_{12}$
- Digestive enzyme
- Other: _____

Foods on the phytonutrient rainbow I ate today (see pages 206–211 in the main book):

- Red: _____
- Red/purple: _____
- Orange: _____
- Orange/yellow: _____
- Yellow/green: _____
- Green: _____
- White/green: _____

My Seven Pillars progress today was:
Great   Good   Fair   Poor

My Daily Journal

_____
_____
_____

Recharge Your Thoughts

Realize if you consume a healthy diet, you will probably get at least 50 percent of the daily values of vitamins and minerals.

WEEKLY UPDATE

General

What positive changes did I notice in my overall health this week?

_____

_____

_____

_____

My weight update: _____

My blood sugar update: _____

My blood pressure update: _____ / _____

My cholesterol level update: _____

Pillar 1: Water

How many ounces of water did I average per day this week?

☐ ☐ ☐ ☐ ☐ ☐ ☐ (one checkbox per 16-ounce bottle)

What adjustments to my beverage intake do I want to make in the coming week? _____

_____

Pillar 2: Sleep and Rest

How many hours of sleep did I average per night this week? _____

What adjustments to my sleep routine do I want to make in the coming week? _____

_____

Pillar 3: Living Foods

How did I excel in choosing living foods this week? _____

_____

_____

How did I depend upon dead foods? _____

_____

_____

What adjustments to my eating habits will I make in the coming week?

_____

_____

Pillar 4: Exercise

What victories did I have in stirring the waters this week? _____

_____

How will I continue to build up my regular exercise schedule in the coming week? _____

_____

Pillar 5: Detoxification

How did I help my body detoxify this week? _____

_____

How can I continue to detoxify and reduce toxic exposure in the coming week? _____

_____

Pillar 6: Nutritional Supplements

How many days this week did I take these supplements?

Whole-food multivitamin: _____ days this week

Phytonutrient powder: _____ days this week

Omega-3 supplement: _____ days this week

Sublingual B_{12}: _____ days this week

Digestive enzyme: _____ days this week

What goals for nutritional supplementation do I have for the coming week? _____

_____

DAY 43

Points to Ponder

Stress can be bad (like experiencing a financial setback), but it can also be good (like getting married). Stress generally falls into two categories: situations that we can control, and situations that are uncontrollable and beyond our skill or knowledge. If we don't learn to manage stress well, it eventually affects every part of us, from the inside out.

Action Step

Complete the stress test on page 127. Completed? ☐ Yes ☐ No

Stress score: _____

Stress level: ☐ Low ☐ Medium ☐ High

Make It Personal

What situations provoke a high level of stress in my life?

_____

_____

_____

How do I usually respond to stressful situations? _____

_____

_____

_____

_____

In what ways has stress affected my health? _____

_____

_____

_____

_____

Daily Checkup

On a scale of 1–10, my stress level today was: _____

Stress factors I faced today: _____

_____

_____

_____

_____

How I coped with these stress factors today: _____

_____

_____

_____

_____

My Seven Pillars progress today was:
　Great　　Good　　Fair　　Poor

My Daily Journal

_____

_____

_____

_____

_____

_____

_____

Recharge Your Thoughts

When you begin to practice mindfulness by enjoying the present moment and to reframe situations by practicing gratitude, your perceptions and reactions change.

DAY 44

Points to Ponder

Mindfulness is training your thoughts to let go of anything other than the present moment. Instead of constantly focusing on getting bigger, better, or more expensive things, be thankful about what you have at the moment, and resist comparing yourself or your possessions with others. Learn to quickly take in what benefits and blessings you have before you, and show (or express) your gratitude regularly.

Action Step

Practice mindfulness by bringing your full attention to every activity you engage in today (at the stop light, at work, on a walk, in conversation, etc). Completed?   ☐ Yes   ☐ No

How did it feel to practice mindfulness in this way? _____

_____

_____

Make It Personal

What preoccupations about the past or future keep me from practicing mindfulness? _____

_____

_____

How do I usually finish the sentence, "I'll be happy when..."?

_____

_____

_____

How can I practice more gratitude in my present moments?

_____

_____

_____

Daily Checkup

On a scale of 1–10, my stress level today was: _____

Stress factors I faced today: _____

_____

_____

_____

_____

How I coped with these stress factors today: _____

_____

_____

_____

_____

My Seven Pillars progress today was:
▢ Great ▢ Good ▢ Fair ▢ Poor

My Daily Journal

_____

_____

_____

_____

_____

_____

_____

Recharge Your Thoughts

To have complete mental and physical health, mindfulness must become a way of life, a continual pattern for practicing relaxation during your day.

DAY 45

Points to Ponder

Reframing is learning to shift your focus away from your present point of view in order to "see" another person or a situation from a new perspective. Like Frankl, imagine yourself coming out free on the other side of your circumstance. Envision all of the positive effects that will result from the situation. The heart's power to bring thoughts back into "sync" is a powerful tool to reframing the mind.

Action Step

Pick a Bible verse that helps you reframe your circumstances, and memorize it this week. Completed?　Yes　No

Which Bible verse did you choose? _____

_____

_____

Make It Personal

What past experiences still haunt me? _____

_____

_____

_____

_____

What positive outcomes can be identified for those experiences?

_____

_____

_____

What scripture verses help reinforce my reframing of these events?

_____

_____

_____

Daily Checkup

On a scale of 1–10, my stress level today was: _____

Stress factors I faced today: _____

_____

_____

_____

_____

How I coped with these stress factors today: _____

_____

_____

_____

_____

My Seven Pillars progress today was:
▢ Great   ▢ Good   ▢ Fair   ▢ Poor

My Daily Journal

_____

_____

_____

_____

_____

_____

_____

Recharge Your Thoughts

Scriptural reframing is one of the most powerful ways to relieve stress.

DAY 46

Points to Ponder

Create a habit of happiness and laughter instead of a habit of worry. When you laugh, it lowers stress hormones and relieves stress. Laughter also boosts the immune system, protects the heart, and improves overall health. Ten belly laughs a day are equivalent to getting a good aerobic exercise workout, and they're the ultimate "stress busters."

Action Step

Watch a TV show or movie that will get you laughing tonight. Completed? ▢ Yes ▢ No

Make It Personal

What makes me laugh? _____
_____
_____
_____
_____
_____

When do I feel the most happy? _____
_____
_____
_____
_____
_____

How many times a day do I usually laugh? _____
_____
_____

Daily Checkup

On a scale of 1–10, my stress level today was: _____

Stress factors I faced today: _____

_____

_____

_____

_____

How I coped with these stress factors today: _____

_____

_____

_____

_____

My Seven Pillars progress today was:
▢ Great ▢ Good ▢ Fair ▢ Poor

My Daily Journal

_____

_____

_____

_____

_____

_____

_____

Recharge Your Thoughts

*Choosing a good attitude doesn't diminish the amount
of suffering in your life or in the world, but it helps
to lighten the load.*

DAY 47

Points to Ponder

When you fail to forgive an offense, you "rehash" that memory and keep yourself trapped in the stress of reliving that moment. Some offenses are real; some are perceived. It all comes down to your perception and whether or not you choose to forgive. Forgiveness is letting go of old hurts and people who wounded you, which will set you free from stress.

Action Step

Identify someone you need to forgive, and verbalize the declaration of release and the prayer of forgiveness toward them on page 128. Completed?   Yes   No

Make It Personal

What grievance stories do I continue to repeat? _____

_____

_____

_____

_____

What physical response does my body give when I rehash these grievances? _____

_____

_____

_____

How can I move toward forgiveness in these areas? _____

_____

_____

_____

Daily Checkup

On a scale of 1–10, my stress level today was: _____

Stress factors I faced today: _____

_____

_____

_____

_____

How I coped with these stress factors today: _____

_____

_____

_____

_____

My Seven Pillars progress today was:
▓ Great ▓ Good ▓ Fair ▓ Poor

My Daily Journal

_____

_____

_____

_____

_____

_____

_____

Recharge Your Thoughts

Forgiving in its simplest form is letting go of old hurts and releasing people and situations into God's hands.

DAY 48

Points to Ponder

Margin, according to Dr. Swenson, is the difference between vitality and exhaustion. I say it is the buffer between feeling overwhelmed and feeling at peace. When you fail to schedule adequate time between events or activities when you do have control, you set yourself up to experience stress. Get off the "do-more-so-I-can-have-more" treadmill! Margin is building time in your schedule, finances, and every area of your life so that you eliminate that unnecessary stress.

Action Step

Make a "to-do" list for what you need to accomplish today, and build plenty of margin between each commitment to de-stress your day. Completed? █ Yes █ No

Make It Personal

How can I relate to the story told at the beginning of the chapter?

_____

_____

_____

How do I need to build better margin into my life (schedule, finances, etc.)? _____

_____

_____

_____

_____

What can I do to begin building this margin? _____

_____

_____

_____

Daily Checkup

On a scale of 1–10, my stress level today was: _____

Stress factors I faced today: _____

_____

_____

_____

_____

How I coped with these stress factors today: _____

_____

_____

_____

_____

My Seven Pillars progress today was:
⬜ Great ⬜ Good ⬜ Fair ⬜ Poor

My Daily Journal

_____

_____

_____

_____

_____

_____

_____

Recharge Your Thoughts

Margin is that buffer between feeling overwhelmed and feeling at peace.

DAY 49

Points to Ponder

Think on good, positive things. Remember that old adage: "Accentuate the positive; eliminate the negative." Practice proper breathing techniques (abdominal breathing), which will help you de-stress. Learn the art of saying no. Do not volunteer or take on more activities than you are capable of handling. Limit the time spent with people who are pessimistic, whiners, or complainers. If you're not careful, they will drain the energy and life right out of you.

Action Step

Take five minutes today to practice the abdominal breathing technique. (See page 256 in the main book.)
Completed?   Yes   No

Make It Personal

In what ways can I bring greater order to my home and work environments? _____

_____

_____

_____

Where do I need to practice the "power of no" in my life?

_____

_____

_____

Which friends and family members have the most positive influence on my life? _____

_____

_____

_____

Daily Checkup

On a scale of 1–10, my stress level today was: _____

Stress factors I faced today: _____

_____

_____

_____

_____

How I coped with these stress factors today: _____

_____

_____

_____

_____

My Seven Pillars progress today was:
◻ Great ◻ Good ◻ Fair ◻ Poor

My Daily Journal

_____

_____

_____

_____

_____

_____

_____

Recharge Your Thoughts

The most important foundation of a stressless life is meditating on the Bible.

DAY 50

Points to Ponder

Jesus is the Prince of Peace and offers you the peace that passes all understanding. The best stress reliever is to pray and begin to learn to cast all your cares on Jesus. Practice trusting in God's Word.

Action Step

Today is your day of jubilee, so thank Him aloud for His goodness! Completed?   Yes   No

Make It Personal

What factors in my life promote peace? _____

_____

_____

_____

_____

_____

What factors keep me from it? _____

_____

_____

_____

_____

_____

How does Jesus offer me peace? _____

_____

_____

_____

_____

_____

Daily Checkup

On a scale of 1–10, my stress level today was: _____

Stress factors I faced today: _____

_____

_____

_____

_____

How I coped with these stress factors today: _____

_____

_____

_____

_____

My Seven Pillars progress today was:
▢ Great ▢ Good ▢ Fair ▢ Poor

My Daily Journal

_____

_____

_____

_____

_____

_____

_____

Recharge Your Thoughts

The most important way to overcome stress is to keep our minds focused on the promises of God's Word and to trust His Word, which brings perfect peace.

WEEKLY UPDATE

General

What positive changes did I notice in my overall health this week?

_____

_____

_____

_____

My weight update: _____

My blood sugar update: _____

My blood pressure update: _____ / _____

My cholesterol level update: _____

Pillar 1: Water

How many ounces of water did I average per day this week?

☐ ☐ ☐ ☐ ☐ ☐ ☐ (one checkbox per 16-ounce bottle)

What adjustments to my beverage intake do I want to make in the coming week? _____

_____

Pillar 2: Sleep and Rest

How many hours of sleep did I average per night this week? _____

What adjustments to my sleep routine do I want to make in the coming week? _____

_____

Pillar 3: Living Foods

How did I excel in choosing living foods this week? _____

_____

_____

How did I depend upon dead foods? _____

_____

_____

What adjustments to my eating habits will I make in the coming
week? _____

_____

_____

Pillar 4: Exercise

What victories did I have in stirring the waters this week?

_____

_____

How will I continue to build up my regular exercise schedule in
the coming week? _____

_____

_____

Pillar 5: Detoxification

How did I help my body detoxify this week? _____

_____

_____

How can I continue to detoxify and reduce toxic exposure in the
coming week? _____

_____

_____

_____

Pillar 6: Nutritional Supplements

How many days this week did I take these supplements?

Whole-food multivitamin: _____ days this week
Phytonutrient powder: _____ days this week
Omega-3 supplement: _____ days this week
Sublingual B$_{12}$: _____ days this week
Digestive enzyme: _____ days this week

What goals for nutritional supplementation do I have for the coming week? _____
_____
_____

Pillar 7: Coping With Stress

On a scale of 1–10, my stress level this week was: _____

Primary stress factors I faced this week: _____
_____
_____
_____
_____
_____

How I'm learning to cope with these stressors: _____
_____
_____
_____
_____

FINAL STEP: ASSESSMENT AND GOALS

What major health improvements have I experienced in the past fifty days? _____

_____

_____

_____

Which of my goals did I reach? (See pages 5–7.)_____

_____

_____

_____

What other goals would I like to continue working toward?

_____

_____

_____

How will I accomplish these? _____

_____

_____

_____

Finally, what things can I offer thankfulness and gratitude to have received from this fifty-day program? _____

_____

_____

_____

_____

_____

_____

APPRECIATION LIST

1. Before you get out of bed in the morning, begin each day by saying, "Today is the best day of the rest of my life. I choose to be happy and to enjoy this day."

2. Make a list of things for which you are thankful. Include:
    a. Your physical being—eyesight, hearing, taste, smell, ability to touch, ability to walk. Be grateful that you have the use of your fingers, hands, arms, legs, and so on.
    b. Modern-day conveniences—a car, running hot water, air conditioning/heater, a working computer, telephone, and so on
    c. Everyday needs—food, a job, water, shelter, and so on
    d. People—spouse, children, relatives, friends, co-workers, and so on (even your pets!)
    e. Nature—flowers, weather, fresh air, or anything in nature that makes you grateful to be alive

3. Review the list daily.

4. Recite it aloud frequently.

5. Update the list periodically.

I AM THANKFUL FOR:

_____

_____

_____

_____

_____

_____

_____

_____

_____

AGREEMENT TO LOSE WEIGHT

Repeat this agreement aloud and with conviction three times a day before meals.

No longer will I only use my willpower to control my eating; instead I will use God's power infused into my willpower through the Holy Spirit. I will crucify my flesh daily and give my body what it needs and not what it craves. I covenant today that no longer will food be my comforter, but the Holy Spirit will be my Comforter.

From this day on, I refuse to pollute my body by eating junk food, sugar, fried foods, and any other food that is unhealthy.

I covenant to exercise at least every other day because I realize that I cannot lose weight and keep it off without exercise.

I CONFESS:

- I want to lose weight and keep it off.
- I deserve to lose weight and keep it off.
- Losing weight is good for me.
- Losing weight is good for others.
- It is safe for me to lose weight and keep it off.
- With the Holy Spirit's help, I will lose weight and keep it off.

_____

YOUR SIGNATURE

BODY MASS INDEX FOR ADULTS TABLE[4]

BMI	Normal						Overweight					Obese									
	19	20	21	22	23	24	25	26	27	28	29	30	31	32	33	34	35	36	37	38	39
Height (inches)	Body Weight (pounds)																				
58	91	96	100	105	110	115	119	124	129	134	138	143	148	153	158	162	167	172	177	181	186
59	94	99	104	109	114	119	124	128	133	138	143	148	153	158	163	168	173	178	183	188	193
60	97	102	107	112	118	123	128	133	138	143	148	153	158	163	168	174	179	184	189	194	199
61	100	106	111	116	122	127	132	137	143	148	153	158	164	169	174	180	185	190	195	201	206
62	104	109	115	120	126	131	136	142	147	153	158	164	169	175	180	186	191	196	202	207	213
63	107	113	118	124	130	135	141	146	152	158	163	169	175	180	186	191	197	203	208	214	220
64	110	116	122	128	134	140	145	151	157	163	169	174	180	186	192	197	204	209	215	221	227
65	114	120	126	132	138	144	150	156	162	168	174	180	186	192	198	204	210	216	222	228	234
66	118	124	130	136	142	148	155	161	167	173	179	186	192	198	204	210	216	223	229	235	241
67	121	127	134	140	146	153	159	166	172	178	185	191	198	204	211	217	223	230	236	242	249
68	125	131	138	144	151	158	164	171	177	184	190	197	203	210	216	223	230	236	243	249	256
69	128	135	142	149	155	162	169	176	182	189	196	203	209	216	223	230	236	243	250	257	263
70	132	139	146	153	160	167	174	181	188	195	202	209	216	222	229	236	243	250	257	264	271
71	136	143	150	157	165	172	179	186	193	200	208	215	222	229	236	243	250	257	265	272	279
72	140	147	154	162	169	177	184	191	199	206	213	221	228	235	242	250	258	265	272	279	287
73	144	151	159	166	174	182	189	197	204	212	219	227	235	242	250	257	265	272	280	288	295
74	148	155	163	171	179	186	194	202	210	218	225	233	241	249	256	264	272	280	287	295	303
75	152	160	168	176	184	192	200	208	216	224	232	240	248	256	264	272	279	287	295	303	311
76	156	164	172	180	189	197	205	213	221	230	238	246	254	263	271	279	287	295	304	312	320

BMI	Extreme Obesity														
	40	41	42	43	44	45	46	47	48	49	50	51	52	53	54
Height (inches)	Body Weight (pounds)														
58	191	196	201	205	210	215	220	224	229	234	239	244	248	253	258
59	198	203	208	212	217	222	227	232	237	242	247	252	257	262	267
60	204	209	215	220	225	230	235	240	245	250	255	261	266	271	276
61	211	217	222	227	232	238	243	248	254	259	264	269	275	280	285
62	218	224	229	235	240	246	251	256	262	267	273	278	284	289	295
63	225	231	237	242	248	254	259	265	270	278	282	287	293	299	304
64	232	238	244	250	256	262	267	273	279	285	291	296	302	308	314
65	240	246	252	258	264	270	276	282	288	294	300	306	312	318	324
66	247	253	260	266	272	278	284	291	297	303	309	315	322	328	334
67	255	261	268	274	280	287	293	299	306	312	319	325	331	338	344
68	262	269	276	282	289	295	302	308	315	322	328	335	341	348	354
69	270	277	284	291	297	304	311	318	324	331	338	345	351	358	365
70	278	285	292	299	306	313	320	327	334	341	348	355	362	369	376
71	286	293	301	308	315	322	329	338	346	353	361	368	375	383	390
72	294	302	309	316	324	331	338	346	353	361	368	375	383	390	397
73	302	310	318	325	333	340	348	355	363	371	378	386	393	401	408
74	311	319	326	334	342	350	358	365	373	381	389	396	404	412	420
75	319	327	335	343	351	359	367	375	383	391	399	407	415	423	431
76	328	336	344	353	361	369	377	385	394	402	410	418	426	435	443

BMI Categories

- Underweight = < 18.5
- Normal weight = 18.5–24.9
- Overweight = 25–29.9
- Obesity = BMI of 30 or greater

LIFE STRESS TEST*

Circle the point value for each event listed that you have experienced in the past two years. When you have circled all the experiences that pertain to you, add the points together. Then use the scale to determine your current life stress level.

Death of a spouse	100
Divorce	73
Marital separation	65
Jail term	63
Death of a close family member	63
Personal injury or illness	53
Marriage	50
Fired at work	47
Marital reconciliation	45
Retirement	45
Change in health of a family member	44
Pregnancy	40
Sex difficulties	39
Gain of a new family member	39
Business readjustment	39
Change in financial state	38
Death of a close friend	37
Change to a different line of work	36
Change in number of arguments with spouse	35
Mortgage over $100,000	31
Foreclosure of mortgage or loan	30
Change in responsibilities at work	29
Son or daughter leaving home	29
Trouble with in-laws	29
Outstanding personal achievement	28
Wife begins or stops work	26
Begin or end school	26
Change in living conditions	25
Revision in personal habits	24
Trouble with boss	23
Change in work hours or conditions	20
Change in residence	20
Change in schools	20
Change in recreation	19
Change in church activities	19
Change in social activities	18
Mortgage or loan less than $30,000	17
Change in sleeping habits	16
Change in number of family get-togethers	15
Change in eating habits	15
Vacation	13
Christmas alone	12
Minor violations of the law	11

* This information was published in *The Journal of Psychosomatic Research*, vol. 11, T. Holmes and R. Rahe, "The Social Readjustments Rating Scales," 213-218, Copyright Elsevier, 1967.

A Declaration to Resolve
Unforgiveness, Resentment, and Bitterness

It is helpful to first picture the person whom you wish to forgive with your eyes closed; then when you can see his/her face, say the name by which you called him/her when he/she first came into your life, and forgive him/her as described below.

Then in the same way, forgive all others, one by one, who have caused you anger, resentment, or pain, or who have caused pain or hurt in those you love. Do not forget to forgive yourself, God, biological parents, step-parents, adopted parents, grandparents, siblings, spouse, ex-spouse(s), children, and any others who have offended you, whether you remember specific events related to each one or not. You can release bitterness with either this affirmation or prayer below.

I choose to forgive [[fill in the name]], *both consciously or subconsciously, for anything that he/she may have done or failed to do. I choose to forgive* [[fill in the name]] *for anything that he/she may have said or failed to say, which in my perception has caused pain in me or anyone else I care about. I also choose to forgive all of those whom I have unforgiveness and resentment toward for any reason. I choose to replace all bitterness with love, joy, and peace.*

Here's a sample prayer:

Father, I acknowledge that I have sinned against You by not forgiving those who have offended me. I also acknowledge my inability to forgive them apart from You. I understand Matthew 6:14–15, which says, "If ye forgive men their trespasses, your heavenly Father will also forgive you: But if ye forgive not men their trespasses, neither will your Father forgive your trespasses." Since Jesus forgave my sins and cancelled my debt by shedding His blood and dying on the cross for me, the least I can do is forgive [[fill in the name]] *and cancel their debt against me. Therefore, with Your help and from my heart, I choose to forgive* [[fill in the name(s)]]. *I release them; they no longer owe me anything. I ask that You bless them and lead them into a closer relationship with You. In Jesus' name, amen.*